TOUCHED BY MADNESS

Seth Finnegan

chipmunkapublishing
the mental health publisher

Seth Finnegan

Published by
Chipmunkapublishing
United Kingdom

http://www.chipmunkapublishing.com

SYNOPSIS

The following collection of fifty poems has been born out of
my own experience of mental illness. I was diagnosed with
Bi Polar disorder in my late thirties and discovered that writing
about it, and other conditions was helpful, even therapeutic.
The aim of the collection is to reach and speak to people, sufferers
or sane alike, giving some insights as to how these illnesses
manifest, covering a wide range of disorders that affect people in
our modern world.

DEDICATION

I wish to thank the following persons for their love and support,
without whom this book could not have been born.
Minnie, my darling wife, carer and researcher extraordinaire
Kirsten Lee, an inspiration wherever she goes
Anne Merrick, a gifted author and motherly mentor
my parents Margaret and Mike for their belief in me
my dear sister Chantal, Julian, Evie, Harriet and Joseph for their
love and support
my second mother Rachel and her great loving family
to Gerry Quaile, my generous buddy and erudite supporter
to the Cumberland Grange poetry group as great friends
to Melbert and Nigel Chambers for their belief and
encouragements
to Judith Thompson, Mick and Chrissy and Exeter Quakers
to Martin, Amy, Matt and Ed at McGahey's Tobacco Co. for
whom
I am the humble poet in residence.
to Judith Maher for her love, prayers and passion for poetry.

THE SPINNING TOP
(Tony Hancock)
The top went madly spinning
Shivering like a flame
Off centre, bent on winning
For itself a greater fame
Each touch of soft persuasion
Pushes it arm's length
Till it shudders with convulsion
Losing balance, slipping strength
And they watch its last rotations
With a hang dog slump and totter
Resigned to abnegations
To the inevitable horror
As it see saws side to side
With a lurch worse than before
So it makes one desperate slide
Then it crashes to the floor

THE LOOKING GLASS

At eight a veiled sun
Trickles the mirror with light

By noon, his arrows break in
Ripping past the curtain

From one till four
The looking glass is bright

By six the scars will heal
Of which I'm certain

Thank God for clouds
That dim his burning eye

The looking glass survives
So why can't I?

TOUCHED BY MADNESS

VINCENT

Vincent has paid for his sweetness
As if brush strokes were scourging his soul
Though the wine and the bread
For the life that he led
Were not able to render him whole

All the stars that were studding his heaven
Were not brighter in force than his eyes
And the colours he chose
Would outlast the world's woes
From a heart never born for goodbyes

How could the brief blast from a barrel
So finish a life that was blest?
For we knew it was sadness
That triggered his madness
Though his soul now forever finds rest

We are waiting in silence for Vincent
Though our hearts are beginning to faint
For the man who could preach
And the hands that could teach
With a canvas, a pallet and paint

SELF HARMER

I do it not for sympathy
I don't know why I do it
All I know, the knife is there
And in my hand, then wild despair
Suddenly envelops me
I slash and then I rue it

My arms bare all the scars
Attempts at suicide
Broken bottles sometimes do
The ones I emptied feeling blue
Then blackness void of stars
With nowhere left to hide

And yet I still survive
With hopeless, haunted eyes
Long shadows yet may overtake
This ugly life I should forsake
This hell hole of a dive
This living I despise

O LET ME HAVE MY LIGHTS

O let me have my lights
I have witnessed their shape
Like fireflies of the nights
Flares, twinkling gems
Diamonds of another world
Inter planetary flames
Pulsing, flashing orbs so great
Our earth is but unschooled
Beacons to the cosmos pearled
By unknown laws have ruled
Ariel fancies to earth's face
Gorgeous scintillating strobes
Varied throughout time and space
Decked with heavens purple robes
Cathedrals starred in lofty heights
O let me have my lights!

Seth Finnegan

TO WHICH I'M GOING
(A suicide by drowning)

I didn't know where I was my love
I didn't know where I was going
My life a mish mash of regrets
A thousand falls, a thousand frets
And seeds insane a sowing

But they found me here again my love
The river keeps on flowing
The bitter nettles by the pass
Do not reproach me on the grass
Do not reproach my going

The moons bright face once spoke my love
That man was full of knowing
He said with every strand of hair
I plucked and brandished in the air
The wind would bless my going

I am not of nothingness my love
Yet had no worth for showing
And now the earth's celestial daughter
Gleams peacefully upon the water
And I undone, am going

O MAN IN THE MOON

O man in the moon
Have you had a good day?
Tell me what you have heard?
Have you something to say?
Overlooking this planet
From the heights where you scan it
I'd be tempted to damn it
If my eyes had turned grey

O man in the moon
Have you ever wept tears?
For the things that you see
Counting all of our years
Overlooking this earth
From the point of its birth
Does it have any worth?
With our follies and fears

O man in the moon
Glowing bright in the sky
Are you glowing for pleasure?
Or just pale with a sigh
For a world turning bad
Does it make the stars mad?
Are you silent or sad?
Turning still a blind eye

O man in the moon
I wish I were you
Cool and recumbent
With a much better view
Are you tempted to chuck it?
Saying "bother them, fuck it!
They have kicked their own bucket,
It's their mess, let 'em stew!"

THE NUMBERS
(Obsessive Compulsive Disorder)

Long after they're dead the numbers come
Trafficking the mind, tightening
Like signs, the ideal thought, dumb
Unspoken, all effort frightening
Whether they land or not they run
As arrows of false lightning

One swallow never made a summer
Fifty thousand seems a curse
Each one chased a figure runner
Replacing hard the one I nurse
I have no rest with each newcomer
And winning leaves me worse

They catch me in the mental loop
The prison of the brains control
The gulls in numbers dive and swoop
I looked for links to give me whole
Connexions, then another troop
More deadly take their toll

I shoot them down, I lay them dead
I watch them rise like wooded posts
They gather, clouds about my head
In multiples, unending hosts
I lie in straights where sunbeams fled
Those thoughts as shipwrecked ghosts

I start, restart each final score
To break the sequence time must crack
The latest image fixed no more
A phantom flies, no trace, no track
Each loss a room, no walls, no floor
Before the mind turns black

TOUCHED BY MADNESS

WHEN THE CLOUDS CAME WITH CROWS

The clouds came with the crows
It was an unfolding of blackness
It was an east wind which carried
Them over my head, o luckless
Ill fated wind, wouldst you had died
Before spring, and the daffodils in golden rows

Had come bursting into sight
But for now, grey clouds bulking
With a sulking wind playing about
My stinging ears and the crows skulking
Sadly, solemnly, screaming their doubt
Through the lingering hours of my protracted night

TO THE DARK LADY I COME

I will give it all up
For the dark lady
She will heal my malady
I drank a bitter cup

I have no real home
I have wandered wild grasses
Some love for pain surpasses
To the dark lady I come

I know many of her sons
Were drowned beneath a keel
Hibernians will feel
The lives which evil shuns

The life I live is rented
Beyond the earth and sea
I will come to the dark lady
God save her, I was tormented

She whispers peace, I hear
Her loving song of hope
The grace by which I cope
For death was often near

I will give it up at length
My days have all been numbered
But now I'm not encumbered
My chains have lost their strength

TROUBLED MIND

Gulls orbit over my head
They are not moon gazing
She that lovelorn, luminous
Locket, lies cradled by stars
I see their difference and distance
To the dark backdrop of night
How endlessly they chime
To unknown rhythms of space
To earth I am fixed in wonder
This same moon and sapphire suns
Glut the vault of Indian skies
Strobe the sands of tropic shores
Could my mind in states aspire
Up to touch those gems of fire
Would I sink at last to find
Nothing more than moon dust here,
Nothing but emptiness I fear?
Would that relieve my troubled mind?

PARIAH

I see men, women, acquaintances
Moving away as dromedaries
From the old stone Quaker house.
They turn away from the path, talking;
I am not in their circle, left sitting
On the wall, too far from their walking.
To them I am a pariah, smoking by the
Heavy black gates. The way in is the
Way out. I've heard provoking thoughts
With wagtails outwitting the shadows
Stealing in by degrees, trapping me
In these quaint circumstances.
The slow moving camels have disappeared.
Now comes the loneliness, sat on the wall.
The man who is down has but nowhere
To fall; but the wind comes with loneliness
Just as I feared.

TERMINAL SICKNESS

The corridor is a lighted runway
But here, no one is taking off
The passengers still carry their baggage
At terminal one where the flight pills
Are dispensed. We gather like chicks
For the evening feed. We all have
Some terminal sickness to be fixed
By the seed. We are flightless birds
Not ready for air, for that is some
Dream to the prisoners of fate shut inside.
In our cells, too high for a hanging
We bed down to the wings of this plane,
This mausoleum transport carrier. And
All of our windows have bars.
Outside there is a blue, black runway
Lit by lamps, set for take off. But it isn't
Happening tonight. We are grounded
Within the stones laid by French prisoners
Here at Wonford House. Only their spirits
Have taken to flight, as we sit in our cabins
Or walk the gangways, waiting for the
Green light, looking at the clouds, watched
By stewards through the peep holes.
We are the goods, the duty frees, tripping out

MAD EYE

I saw a woman in Torquay
In the high street, near the sea
Her eye was blind and fixed on me

Its colour mottled, misty grey
We laughed, but what the eye would say
Is blindness comes at close of day

Pupiless, the eye opaque
Was tearless with the words it spake
And said the world you must forsake

The world of bitter works, regrets
The world of dirt, disease and debts
The world of sickness, cigarettes

Passing us were many folk
Between the words, between the smoke
But that mad eye so clearly spoke

I looked above her head, the blue
Sky with a bright sun bursting through
Was sanity where freedom flew

But o that eye midst briefest gladness
Looked at me with hidden sadness
Speaking with a mote of madness

TOUCHED BY MADNESS

GULLS BY DAY AND NIGHT

The gulls by day are demented
Pillaging bins and hungry for scrap
Perhaps like many they are tormented
Yet in the midnight blue, the trap

Of earth they loose with silent wings
And glide the cool, untroubled air
Above the world's sad sickenings
To make me wish that I were there

Somewhere lost in beauties flight
Held within a gentle breeze
Swallowed in the depths of night
Crying not for wealth of ease

And so it is I weep inside
To be like gulls which seem to find
An answer in the winds they bide
The winds which vex my troubled mind

Seth Finnegan

GHOSTS WITHIN THESE CORRIDORS

Up and down the deck we go
Cabin doors creaking in the wind
No one in the crows nest watching
No one to the steering pinned

Now I know we have no captain
Only stars to plot our course
Up and down we tread the gangways
Ghosts within these corridors

We scan horizon points for land
Twixt the moons and suns which change
Nothings fixed upon this ship
Each and every day is strange

And all the sirens that we hear
Bring some poor wretch to walk these floors
At cuckoo time when all resemble
Ghosts within these corridors

TOUCHED BY MADNESS

Touched by madness
Singed with sadness
Where's the pill
Returning gladness?

Damn these devils
Wild with revels
Where's the lithium
Which levels?

Brings me round
Makes me sound
Brings me back
To solid ground

Highs are cheap
My mind must keep
A grip on health
Before I sleep

Seth Finnegan

GREAT SOUL

Am I mad because I
Do not comply, conform?
To man made parameters, why
Should this be the norm?

My brain thinks clear, but in pain
Shackled by dull convention
The rules so silly and vain
From which I make my abstention

And because I am singled out
A lunatic from the word go
Do you have a lingering doubt
That right is the status quo?

My brain only needs a pill
To make of it beautiful art
And sane is my beautiful will
And in my great soul, what heart!

THE LITTLE ROSE BUD

I am a small bud
I am red from my birth
Let me hide myself
In my pleasant greenery

I have felt the cold whip
Of the wind in her strength
In secret you must find my good
In my native, warm earth

With dew drops I mingle
Untroubled by thorns
My petals complete, but folding
Uncrushed and at rest

I have seen the bright dawns
Solitary and single
Fragile, always holding
Living hours that test

All that's wild and free
About my palaces no less
My rain washed head
My sun blanched face

Speak peace most tenderly
If near me you tread
Water with tears my place
Smile with your gentleness

THE KEYS

I saw a man on his landing
Go back and forth, to and fro
He was locked by OCD
He could go in, he had a key
I wanted to call out to break
His sad midnight routine
He may have spooked, I held my peace
Only the white spectres of space
The gulls with effortless ease
Were scribing the black evening
Feathered quills to the ink of night
Writing their names in the air
Only they have keys to freedom there

SHE TAKES MY HANDS

There is a woman, she takes my hands
She leads me at her own sweet will
She leads me so, for I am ill
She takes me for she understands

It is because she is alert
To some strange need that she can see
And so it is she must lead me
Because it is my mind is hurt

And when she does, I have no notion
But to follow where she goes
Like a stream that ebbs and flows
So she gets my true emotion

And all I give are daffodils
Because she knows my mental pain
She never takes my hand in vain
To leave me free of mental ills

OLD VOICES

The rain floods me like a flower
When for its fall, the voices cease
It is the release of heavenly power
And then comes my peace

But I am mad for familiar voices
They come like nails hard hitting again
With all known points of reference, choices
Tormenting my brain

As dogs they bark, like cats they mew
They spew such poison that none can hear
They are false like old phantoms which ever renew
To my innermost ear

But the rain seems to wash them away like a smut
The noises of voices which batter my head
Yet when the clouds clear for me there's a but
The old voices instead

The soft silent drill of the rain turns to snow
White as the belly and wings of a gull
Perhaps it will stifle those tongues and let go
The rage in my skull

But the snows will all melt and the earth will appear
And the light will then harden, the gulls will take heart
And cry, shrill dementedly, then what I fear
The old voices shall start

THE BEAUTIFUL, IMPERFECT ME
(Body Dysmorphia accepted)

I am an image that changes
It is full of weird contradictions
It constantly rearranges

There are no standard conditions
My hair is lank, my skin goes red
Are these odd things all in my head?

Others do not see at all
The way I see myself, it's true
And really I don't want them to

I hate the way I look so fat
I loathe myself for being small
Too conscious of my image that

I bury something deep inside
The soul of me, I know it's sad
For really, am I all that bad?

Forever must I so deride
The soul that others love to see
The beautiful, imperfect me?

I AM ILL

I am the voice of the drowning
The sun downing souls of dementia
Their mercy shall be no censure
Out of mind, till the glad morning
But my morning comes without sun
I am undone

I am pricked by my past happenings
Looted and spoilt for leisure
My peace has been took with my treasure
Which I search in my rude beginnings
My only comfort comes with the night
Relaxing the fight

I am hard pushed by my OCD
Its grip is continual friction
My life is a vast contradiction
A desert that's swallowing me
An ocean that's drowning me still
I am ill

TOUCHED BY MADNESS

THIS SIDE OF TOWN

I am the blitzed in flesh and bone
But above this bombed out mind
The wreckage and ruins still standing
Past episodes I've left behind
The memories like winds that moan
Speak clear but voice no understanding

Like soldiers now we are surviving
Others sail on like the birds
We do not fly with fractured wings
We hardly speak with broken words
As smouldering flax we need reviving
Who speaks the tongue of sufferings?

The priests and doctors gave us up
For prayers and pills that say no more
That we are now beyond their care
Who once came knocking at death's door
And drank the dregs, a bitter cup
Who can but only stand and stare

What is this roller coaster ride
Bipolar gives to troubled hearts?
Please stop this trip that's up and down
Before the next one badly starts
I only want the sunny side
From where I live this side of town

IT ISSUES FROM THE MOTHER

They've tried to isolate the gene
For manic depression
They think it issues from the mother
The code that makes the deep impression
I could have guessed it so my brother
For all that I have known and seen

She always was a mixed up hen
That mother mine, the mental sort
Digging blackheads from my face
And rowing daily just for sport
O take me to another place
To where they can't fuck up again

And now that they are old and grey
My folks who've tried to put it right
They don't know sanity from madness
How mad it is when parents fight
How children cop the worst of sadness
From having screwed up yesterday

SUICIDE

Some have written into their DNA
Their suicide, the final day
The final word, their own way out
Hung between black clouds of doubt
Despise not this, their sad demise
They couldn't see life through your eyes

I too have sat a lonely rock
Have felt the sea sprays shivering shock
Have tried in vain to trace the sun
Could not find smiles in anyone
Felt vanity with lonely breath
Saw edens through the veil of death

Do not despise their passing through
They didn't know what else to do
They couldn't sing their songs on earth
For blind were they to their own worth
So lullaby their lives at last
Beyond the torrid oceans blast

Seth Finnegan

MULTIPLE PERSONALITY DISORDER

I don't know who I really am
Once I was Susan, then I was Steve
Sometimes I don't give a damn
I only know what I believe

Perhaps I hide in masks I wear
Putting on the latest front
I want to make you stop and stare
A pop star with the latest stunt

And then I slip into myself
Alone, afraid against the wall
And there I sit upon the shelf
Where no one looks at me at all

TOUCHED BY MADNESS

MY REASONS WHY
(Bi Polar Reflections)

My eyes were pits of despair
Serenity would come with nights
My madness couldn't bide the lights
But peace was with the midnight air
Locked to the stars my soul would stare

Up and down I could scale
The blue, blackness of space
To unknown constellations trace
The stars, my friends which never fail
My mother moon, my holy grail

Birds at dusk relieved my ears
My thoughts, whatever such are worth
I loved the little birds of earth
Calming, charming out dark fears
Yes, more so with the coming years

We may not know our time to die
But let I pray, my final breath
Be not a song which dies with death
The birds, the stars have heard my cry
Yet need not know the reasons why

Seth Finnegan

BUDS OF REASON

The wind is snarling at the buds
The flush of thoughts lie still
The wind will then sleep until
The storm stirs emotional moods

Then when spring works warm enchantment
When my head is happy again
The blossom will shed its disdain
To flutter pink bells on my casement

It is only the tree blight I fear
Moulding and rotting my fruits
To fungus cerebral roots
The thoughts that are trapped in my head

Without thoughts, without blossoms I die
With the greening ideas on the bough
Don't let the wind take me, not now
That I'm ready for sunbeams and sky

WHEN THE EVENING DARKENS

Unpardoning clouds open, cold
Rain all day. There is a schism
In the sky, which isn't seen.
It is too grey for ideas to bud,
Too freezing for buds to spread.
The ocean rages under starless vaults,
Like a frozen wave the hotel windows
Face me untenanted, black,
Inscrutable. People move on through
The drizzle and dampness talking.
Car tyres sizzle the wet tarmac.
Industry, commerce, continues.
I heard they are cutting more trees,
More pulp and more fires to burn.
My own leaves have turned with
The winds, trying vainly to shield my buds.
Only when the wind and traffic dies
Like excrement flushed down the toilet
And the evening darkens, I dream again
Of a place without people to spoil it.

HE WAS A NUT

It's fair to say he was a nut
A religious nut it's true
But I loved him more
For the mental flaw
Though he didn't have a clue
Caught in religions rut

For the sad old world of silly men
And women lacking charm
Do more by hate
To aggravate
As hypocrites that harm
I've seen it time and again

"I'm all right Jack!" that's the word
"Bugger the nutters!" they say
They drive big cars
Ignore the stars
The world is their only way
So fly them, dear nut, like a bird
Rise up with thy beads, fly away!

APOPHENIA

I have come to love Apophenia
She gives me sweet patterns
Sometimes I miss her connexions
But that's not what really matters

She fixes me with sugar grains
It's then I see the stars
With constellations salts my plate
Turns tissues into flowers

Superstitiously I love
The way she turns my head
The rain floats diamonds from the sky
To jewel the path I tread

She dances in the silver pearls
Of dewdrops on the grass
Then blows a blossom on my brow
To let my madness pass

I walk in funny ways to trace
Pink petals at my feet
To tread the green of uncut grass
When walking down the street

To catch the sheet of summer sky
Which clouds have not yet cloaked
And I the draught horse to her plough
Am beautifully yoked

TWO LINES

When two lines meet
Psychosis ceases
At least to the naked eye
But the illness will belie
And break me in pieces
On any old street

It did long years past
In a dark episode
I wrestled the arm
Of the law causing harm
To myself on some road
So weak from a fast

Of forty hard days
Then time in gaol
With paper clothes that itch
Bi polar is a glitch
And madness was my bale
To pass that phase

Then lithium carbonate
Straddling the lines
Blurred as they often did
Bi polar blows its lid
When you don't know the signs
You're in hell of a state

Then they find your range
And you chill in time
Sharing each other's shoes
Hard put to answer clues
That this had reason or rhyme
Those two lines are strange

BRICK SHIT

Some bricks have the sea gull shit
That's just where the excrement fell
There's no rhyme nor reason to it
They fly with grace but scream like hell

Another child is shaken to death
Bears are caged, it makes me mad
And others from their birth to breath
Collect water from a stream gone bad

Others wounded from a blitz
Of bombs are treated for their scars
Whilst wealth dines daily at the Ritz
And those with fame are called the stars

And one who belches spite and malice
Raising buildings to the ground
Sits within his onion palace
Guilty, but he won't be found

The world is mad, or is it me?
Confounded by its wicked tricks
The grinning gulls are sailing free
And still keep shitting on the bricks

Seth Finnegan

WOMAN ON THE FLOOR

I saw a woman on the floor
Pulling at her wretched hair
Screaming with a wild despair

I saw her sat up in the bed
Like a spectre, white as hoar
Hands upon her troubled head

Working out the reason why
Her husband left her for another
Pity her, that wretched mother

Madness floating in her eye
Hurting from that hard rejection
Hopeless in that dark dejection

Scrabbling on the terracotta
Look no more for there is not a
Loving hand to help but me

But this alone can't set her free
Replacing tears with happy smiles
Tormented on the kitchen tiles

I read the psalms, I sometimes prayed
Her through the hours of deep depression
Heard the voice change in regression

Till girl she was, again afraid
Alone in silence, like a seed
That's dead from unrequited need

TOUCHED BY MADNESS

THE LOVELY GIRL

The girl with Down's Syndrome
Isn't ill and isn't dull,
Not like the sour faced shoppers,
No, thrice no, she's beautiful

With gorgeous, healthy, chestnut hair
And skin fair like a rose no less,
Waiting tables, like a child,
Unconscious of her loveliness

I'd like to tip her if I could,
My thought for that so agonizes,
But I am skint and do not wish
To be someone who patronizes

A man comes in and seats himself,
They greet, she sits down with her phone;
Relieved for once of gentle duties,
For now the staff leave her alone

And I am ill with hidden sickness,
Having walked a hundred towns,
And pity still the sour, grey faces,
Not the lovely girl with Down's.

ANXIETY

I do not need your piety
Or dull faced sad propriety
It isn't due to dietary
Disorders or ubiety
Or lack of sound sobriety
Or interests of variety
Which gives me notoriety
That only breeds dubiety
And want of inner satiety
It could be the absurdity
Of life in its entirety
That gets at my velleity
And probes my incredulity
To compound my perplexity
Which aggravates necessity
For comforts of propinquity
It could be God, the Deity
It might be just society
But at my most extremity
That makes me mad and crotchety
And often rather fidgety
Depleting my alacrity
It's peace in all its paucity
I suffer from anxiety

TOUCHED BY MADNESS

FINAL VERSE

I contemplate dying, but how and when
Shall I finish it all and pull the plug?
To my own demise, it plays again
Like a record drowning out the glug
That's already started, but how shall it be
The final verse, the end of me?

Perhaps I'll try hanging, it doesn't take long
To set it all up, it's tempting to try it
Jumping's too messy, and drowning's all wrong
And guns are illegal, there's nowhere to buy it
Maybe barbiturates mingled with drink
Is the better way to top the brink!

I have a dear sister in Switzerland
I could stay with her, sign with a physician
They can give you a pill on a patients demand
It's legal out there, all you need is permission
Then into the mountains to fall in the snow
Can you think of a nicer, more neat way to go?

Seth Finnegan

O WHAT BETTER PLACE FOR A NEAT SUICIDE

O Switzerland, the land of free choices
Old men in corduroys, braces and voices
Of yodelling, echoing down from the mountains
And meadows of edelweiss, laughter like fountains
From dairymaids, goat herders, Switzerland's pride
O what better place for a neat suicide!

A pill for the passion and into the snow
Falling face downwards where no one can know
Ending it painlessly, pure, fresh and clean
A snowdrift to cover the tracks that have been
A green spread of grasses way down the hillside
O what better place for a neat suicide!

I could go in a moment and register there
With a doctor, then go in the fresh mountain air
They assist you, it's legal, it's how it should be
It's my life, nobody shall take it from me!
A bitter sweet pleasure, the white snow shall hide
O what better place for a neat suicide!

OLD ROADS, NEW FACES

Old roads and new faces
And the green grasses of hope
Flutter a silent promise to the year
How do depressives live or cope
How do they raise a smile of cheer?
When labelled all lost cases
We see things with a different slant
We're different, so they say
There's things we do which others can't
Our Springs begin in May
It's only that we're catching up
We started with a bitter cup
We tread the old roads with the rest
We're laughing when we cry
You witnessed us when down, depressed
When clouds had choked our sky
But life is good twixt us and you
When suns of hope come bursting through

Seth Finnegan

THE WINDOWS OF THE SOUL

The windows of the soul
Have been too used to seeing
Distortions like a hall of mirrors
As men think so they are
The way I thought became my errors
And so I loathe my imperfections
My very being
Can you help me see my ears
My mouth, my putty nose?
With love's perceptions
Then if you can go that far
The self shall settle whole
And gladly see itself
To put to bed my woes
For new found worth is wealth
Forgetting all my tears

FALLEN LEAVES

Some never notice leaves which fall
Not so much within the town
With eyes forever gazing down
To phones on call
As flecks of paint in yellow spots
They never see in parking lots
Or scattered in the shopping mall
Though banished be by winds
That stroke, the maple tree
The mighty oak
They fall like dreams
Which once awoke
The hearts of broken men
And as you see them strewn around
The pavements grey, without a sound
Tread carefully with courage new
To make dreams come again

Seth Finnegan

WHY DO YOU JUDGE ME?

Why do you judge me?
I am small, of no account
I watch the giddy gadfly
On his luckless quest
A mirror to my own
Midst autumn change
Yet I live
The wind that so bullied
The green leaves, dies
And with it the whisper
Of promises unfulfilled
The dead leaves were not killed
They just burnt out like filaments
Yellow, orange, red , they formed
Mosaics to the mind
They once loved the trees
Like a church they said
But if they die for want
Of love and light, and
The sacramental mystery
Why with things so great and sad
Do you still judge me?

THE CROSSING (A POEM OF AN INTENDED SUICIDE)

I am crossing over now
To the dark side of unchartered space
I have seen the Plough
Will gladly say I have bartered
This earth of salt and grass
For the jewels which I shall pass

A half moon hooks the sky
The gems of night blaze forth
The sleeping cattle lie
On fields which gave them birth
Orion swings his belt
Proud Venus starts to melt

The issue of the stars
Come calling to the stones
They clock eternal hours
O'er Neolithic bones
And home is overhead
The path which I must tread

I'm crossing with the wind
Which stirs the watchful owl
This heaven fills my mind
The foxes start to prowl
They shall not find me here
Eternity draws near

KLEPTOMANIA

He takes for any reason known to man
He thinks the social fabric let him down
He writes his name revengefully through town
With every chance to steal things if he can
Why wasn't he picked up at school
Or in his early teens
Why could his parents never stop
Their loveless ways by any means?
So the Joe they know, breaks all the rules
And takes for fun, or just for thrills
They mark him down with all the fools
And label him with mental ills
(Conclusion)
Can the leopard change his spots? They say
Like leopards treat him not
He only wants what you have got
Which life once took away.

BRIGHT BALLOONS

We are grasping at small bits of string
Bright balloons which embody our dreams
But the wind is too strong with its swing
And they run like streams

Out to unprophesied seas
Past the bluff suns yellow eye
Picking them off by degrees
As the others fly

Beyond reach, beyond touch, out of view
Only a seed thought returns
To awake in our heads something new
Which the wind only spurns

But without dreams the mind only gropes
For a shadow of meaning and then
We start blowing up new balloons for hopes
On the old strings again

Seth Finnegan

BRIGHT PETALS
(A poem about Dementia)

Pale is the pink on the blossom tree
So delicate and pale is she
To the wind she offers up her arms
What calms her now?

Flagrantly the lime green willow
Hangs her head without a pillow
Rain stung, with the washing of winds
Behind, above, below

Some daffodils on bending stalks
Struggle, stoop, the wind still walks
Are they no less afflicted here?
Does fear for them exist?

For these things set to stand the day
Of troubled winds, do flowers say?
"Depart and leave my fragile earth
Of ruby worth, desist!"

I see wild seeds are blown around
In violence without a sound
They fall and die, yet perish not
Spared from the fate of nettles

And when I see my lover so
She slips with smiles and letting go
Is harder than she'll ever know
To share with her bright petals

TOUCHED BY MADNESS

BROKEN HEARTS COULD HARDLY SPEAK

We with broken hearts could hardly speak
Our thoughts we sobbed out on the gutters grey
Oppressions in the system made us weak
Intimidations taught us not to say
Quite how we were and how our lot was doing
Till paths of hope seemed little worth pursuing

The only thing which kept us going places
Were thoughts that somehow sunlight follows rain
We grasped at straws for just some smiling faces
To make us feel some sense of worth again
Then in our corners dark but undenied
We broke like precious vases, there we cried

We saw but little light, the darkness keeping
Our company, our eyes were red and sore
All shades of blue was what we knew with weeping
With promises that promised nothing more
To flee the poor man's grind is what we're after
To see the sun and hear the children's laughter

Like Hannah in the temple so we poured
Our hearts out, sad words twisted on the tongue
At times we felt our voices God ignored
And as the psalmist cried "O Lord how long?"
We wait reply to prayers, press on, look up
The world our priest, which sees a bitter cup

With rapture songbirds trill the morning air
With comforts hear them close all days of weathers
I wonder at the rhapsodies they share
Worlds of joy in little bones and feathers
Small needs perhaps, O let my soul be quickened
To catch their happiness for just one second

ANHEDONIA

Have you been to Anhedonia?
Where the sea mists border the brain
There is never a sun
And the stars have all run
To the edges of darkness again

Her forests are dense and condemning
Her trees black as tar in each line
And as the moon pales
Their branches like nails
Scratch heaven again for a sign

Anhedonia is fruitless and barren
And the banks of her rivers are dry
With grey shadowed eyes
Each citizen cries
With a desperate look to the sky

The children have left Anhedonia
They were spirited off on the wind
And the sound of their laughter
Was swallowed soon after
By the grasses they left far behind

The streets of Anhedonia lie ruined
The paths of her peace withered all
And they wander instead
Like the damned of the dead
With no hands helping hands when they fall

TOUCHED BY MADNESS

One pass leads you to Anhedonia
No ticket's return coming back
It's a trip through the brain
On a cold, empty train
Where the stars are engulfed into black

Seth Finnegan